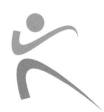

PHYS|CAL F|TNESS

5BX 11-Minute Plan for Men

First published in Great Britain in 2015 by:

BX Plans Ltd
Remus House
Coltsfoot Drive
Peterborough
PE2 9BF
United Kingdom

Contents

5BX 11-Minute Plan For Men

Foreword

When did you last have to walk a long distance, or go on a long walk for pleasure? These days we are much more likely to go on wheels, whether our own or by public transport. Doing less exercise means it is harder to keep fit, especially if you don't want to spend time and money on gym membership. You may not be interested in body building, but nevertheless want to be healthy. If that is you, then this exercise plan is for you; it's the solution to your situation.

The programme of exercises in this book are designed to ensure you reach the peak of physical fitness for you, no matter what state you begin in or how old you are. The exercises are designed to take as little time and space as possible. They are ideal for those of you who lead a relatively sedentary life, perhaps who live in a city, and for those who are becoming aware of things such as a little middle-aged spread or the time pressures of work, but who do not want to have to make a huge effort to change.

It may look like a lot of exercises, but the system is graded and to begin with the exercises are quite gentle and simple. You don't move on until you can complete these sections with ease in the allocated time. How fast you progress through the course depends on you. A reasonable level of fitness will be reached in easy steps, without excessive effort, and all you spend is a little energy for a few minutes daily. You will not become an Olympic athlete overnight, but you will become as fit as you need to be. If you want to get fit, look fit and stay fit, then this programme is for you.

5

Introduction

Why you need to be fit

Scientific researchers have discovered that if you are physically fit, your stamina is improved and you're better able to endure fatigue for longer periods than someone who is not as fit. You will have a healthier heart and you will be better equipped to deal with stress. The research has found that there is a positive relationship between being fit and better mental alertness without any nervous tension.

Remember that if your abdominal muscles are weak then your stomach will sag, and if your back muscles aren't strong enough you are more likely to have back pain.

There are lots of reasons why you are better off if you are fit. People will be able to see you are fit, and you will feel better in yourself. Doing exercise on a regular basis improves both your appearance and your sense of self-worth. You only have one life and, if you want to enjoy it to the fullest, then get fit.

Controlling your weight

Weight control is about altering the relationship, or ratio, of body tissues – you want to decrease the amount of fat and improve your muscles. This will mean controlling your diet as well as partaking in an exercise regime. It isn't necessarily about eating less, but more about eating better.

Whatever we eat the body deals with. Some is stored, some is used as fuel and the rest discarded. The body stores extra calories, or fuel, as fat. A simple analogy to illustrate: If you overfill a bucket, the spare water simply spills out. The body doesn't work like that with calories. It takes in and retains whatever it is offered, however much that is in excess of what it needs, so it is logical that the more you eat the more you will store, unless you use some up by doing exercise.

So, for example, eat 4,000 calories and only use up 2,500, and the surplus 1,500 calories will be stored as fat. Every 3,500 calories consumed in excess of what is used will result in a pound of weight gained – half a bag of sugar. That soon adds up to needing a bigger size in clothing.

On the other hand, when you exercise, calories are burned off. Energy spent in this way will improve your muscle tone. Muscle, however, weighs slightly more than fat, so although your shape may improve, you will not necessarily lose weight. But muscle weight is weight which is useful.

If you do want to lose weight then the researchers tell us that you can do this most effectively by careful eating combined with exercise.

Being fit to live by living to be fit

The aim of this book is to describe how you can use both exercise and diet to achieve a desired level of fitness. Just try out these exercises and make them part of your daily routine, and you will soon notice a positive difference with very little extra effort.

As well as these exercises, you could try simple things, such as getting off the bus or train a stop earlier than usual and walking at a fairly fast pace that extra bit of your journey. Whenever you can, walk instead of riding or driving, and climb the stairs instead of getting frustrated waiting for the lift or using the escalator.

Even drying after the bath or shower can be turned into a mini exercise if you dry yourself briskly, rather than rubbing gently.

Many of us spend hours sitting at a desk, but even then you can exercise by becoming aware of your posture. Sit up as straight as you can, without slouching or rounded shoulders. To strengthen the muscles in your shoulders and arms, place both palms flat on the desk. Bend your elbows and then push hard downwards to try and lift yourself right out of the chair for a few seconds. Doing this just three times a day takes hardly any time at all, but is just one example of using time wisely to improve your fitness.

When standing or sitting, pull in those abdomen muscles and hold them tense for about 6 seconds – count one elephant, two elephants etc., up to six, before relaxing the muscles.

Check up on yourself from time to time during the day. How is your posture? Can it be improved?

Physical wellbeing and fitness

Most of the human body is made up of muscles, bones and fat. You have 639 different muscles and each one:

- can produce force which can be measured
- can store energy so that it can have endurance
- can shorten itself or contract at various speeds – a process described as contraction rates
- can be stretched and then recoiled – this is because of its elasticity.

These four qualities or abilities of your muscles are referred to as muscle power. In order to function to their maximum ability the muscles need fuel on a continuous basis. It is the job of the circulatory system to carry energy in the form of oxygen from the lungs and other necessities from the digestive system. The powerful heart works to force the blood carrying these things around the body to where they are needed, a process known as proving organic power.

It follows that the efficiency and capacity of your body depends upon this organic power, that is the way in which your muscles are developed, combined with organic power and regular exercise. The level to which this muscular development can take place depends upon your body type, the food eaten and whether or not you have some medical condition which might impede it. The amount of rest and sleep you have are also involved. You can only consider yourself to be physically fit when your body is working at its most efficient level.

How fit could you be?

The genes you have inherited, combined with your health, will determine the level of fitness you can ultimately reach, that is your individual physical capacity. In most cases, however hard we train, we will never match the fitness of top Olympic athletes. We are just not made that way, but that does not mean you can't improve on your present state. The level at which you can perform right now is referred to as your 'acquired state', acquired, that is, through the physical acts you already perform as part of daily life.

Like a car engine, your body can perform efficiently at well below its maximum effort. Just as a car uses more fuel if driven at constant high speeds, than if driven at 30-50mph – well below what it is ultimately capable of – in the same way, your body has a better energy to work ratio if it is worked at a level below its full capacity.

It you want to avoid wasting energy you need to have a level of physical capacity which is higher than you need on a daily basis. Taking part in a regime of regular physical exercise will help you to achieve this. The capacity will increase as you quite gradually increase the load required from your muscles and body systems. Exercise increases both your endurance and stamina, and you build up stores of energy to use at your leisure.

Resting, relaxing and revitalising

Your body needs exercise, but just as necessary is rest and relaxation. However, we don't all need the same amount of sleep, and you will know what you need to feel refreshed and revitalised.

If you want to sleep really well, try these tips.

- Keep the bedroom as dark as possible. You can line your curtains with blackout material relatively cheaply and it really makes a difference if you have street lights outside, if there is a full moon, or during those early summer sunrises.
- Try not to take all your problems to bed with you, but instead think calm, positive thoughts.
- Taking mild exercise, such as walking the dog, before bed can help.
- If you are hungry, don't have a big meal, but a light snack and a warm drink will help.

If you don't relax mentally then this will affect your physical body in the form of muscular and organic tension.

Such tension can be reduced considerably if you can teach yourself to deliberately relax muscle groups. For instance, you can relax arm muscles by holding your arms out in front of you and making tight fists and then relaxing them so that your hands are floppy. Do something similar with other muscle groups, stretching and then relaxing and wriggling to relaxation.

Mentally relax by deliberately thinking of relaxing things and ignoring thoughts about anything that has troubled you in the day. Also, taking gentle exercise, such as going for a walk or playing a round of golf, will ease both physical and mental tensions.

Exercise and your heart

Your heart is a muscle and benefits from exercise. There is no evidence to suggest that the heart can be harmed by a sensible exercise regime if it is appropriate for your age and physical state. Instead, it is likely to improve your heart health and that of the major blood vessels. Even after a heart attack, mild exercise is recommended by the medical fraternity, and for the healthy heart there are many benefits. If you are fit there will be a smaller increase in your pulse rate under physical stress, and also your heart rate will return to normal levels more quickly afterwards. A fit heart pumps more blood at rest and can increase this volume when needed. It is more efficient than an unfit heart and the small blood vessels which feed it function better. Such an efficient cardiovascular system will be able to carry oxygen and food to the muscles more effectively, as well as being able to recover better after a period of exercise.

A word of caution

Before undertaking any strenuous exercise regime, anyone with any existing medical condition should seek advice from their doctor. Depending upon the condition, particularly if it is related to the heart, intense exercise could make matters worse.

Strength, endurance and exercise

You can increase the strength and endurance of your body by undertaking exercise. Both the muscles and organs will benefit. You do need to exercise the whole body. Your arm muscles will not benefit if you concentrate only on your leg muscles, so there needs to be a balanced regime of exercise.

Your muscle strength can be measured by checking the amount of force it can exert. This depends on two things – the number of muscle fibres in use and how often the muscles receive impulses from the nervous system.

Strength goes along with endurance. The latter is about being able to keep up muscular contraction, or to repeat a particular action a number of times, such as being able to do ten leg lifts and gradually increasing this number with practice.

The fuel needed to do this, food and oxygen, is carried to the muscle by the bloodstream and this in turn depends upon the strength and efficiency of the cardiovascular system, as well as its ability to carry away waste materials as needed.

If your body is not used, it will deteriorate. If you have ever broken a bone you will have seen and felt, when a plaster cast is eventually taken off, that the muscles underneath are thinner and weaker than they were before the break happened. Unlike a machine, which will wear out with use and eventually break down, the body actually improves the more it is used. Therefore, if you exercise sensibly, more than is needed for basic everyday life, your body will increase in strength, efficiency and in its ability to endure; and your sense of wellbeing, as well as your appearance of health, will both be enhanced.

Caution

If you are in any doubt at all about your body's ability to undertake these exercises do see your doctor first and ask their advice. Also remember that you should start slowly and gradually increase your exercises, especially if you are over 65 years of age.

Your appearance

The appearance of your body depends to a large extent upon the frame, the skeleton beneath. This is something that obviously cannot be changed through exercise, you can, however, alter the amount of fat you have and the firmness of your muscles.

We all need some fat if our bodies are to function properly. As well as softening the bony contours, fat works to control body temperature at a constant level and also acts as a form of storage. As well as a layer of fat beneath the skin, each organ is lined and covered with fat and it also interlaces the muscles.

Except in the case of a few very particular medical conditions, most of us only gain too much fat if we eat more calories than we need and do not work them off.

As well as the amount of fat, muscles are also important in giving the body its appearance. When we are young our muscles have natural tone, but as we age this tone can weaken and be lost. The less exercise we do, the more likely it is that muscles will become flabby and soften. If not used, they weaken and shrink.

Because muscles are so important to your bodily appearance, it is important that you are in control of them by combining a healthy diet with exercise. For example, a thigh may be a certain measurement, but it can be made up mostly of fat or of muscle, two very different things. The difference is up to you. A word of warning: don't confuse good muscle tone with obvious bulky and ugly muscles. The exercises in this book are not designed to produce a body builder's body, but simply to give you the firm muscles you need.

Diet

Often, when a person finds they have gained some weight, the automatic reaction is to go on a diet, sometimes quite a stringent regime. If that is what you intend to do, then research one that will best suit you and your lifestyle, allowing you the time and commitment to follow it effectively. Remember, a diet should not be fast.

Usually, fat is added to the body at quite a slow rate. Therefore, you cannot expect it to come off quickly. Sensible and effective weight loss takes time. A crash diet lasts for a relatively short time, and as soon as the diet is over, invariably, you return to your previous ways, and the fat piles on once more. Instead, make slight changes in your diet, ones you can keep up over time. Cut down on the sugar in your drinks and eat one less slice of bread, or use a smaller cereal bowl and have one less drink in the bar. You will hardly notice the change after a day or two, but it will bring results over time if combined with sufficient exercise, because over a month or so you will have eaten hundreds, if not thousands, of calories less than you might have done. By the time you have reached your desired weight the changes you have made will be a natural part of your daily routine, and so you are less likely to slip back into old habits.

Sports and other activities make a useful contribution

A balanced diet requires a little of everything and, in the same way, you need to balance physical activities so that all parts of your body are exercised. No one sport is likely to do this however, and it may be that your abdomen and back, arms and shoulders, legs or circulatory system are not getting their fair share. But you can't take part in every sport – there is neither the time, the perceived need nor the inclination. For most people the practical answer is to take part in some sport alongside a programme of balanced exercises. The exercises described in this book make up such a programme, and it only takes 11 minutes each day.

Being sensible about exercise

We have all heard about 'the burn' or exercising until it hurts. What nonsense. Pain is not necessary in order to get fit. To avoid any pain or discomfort when exercising:

- Always warm-up appropriately first before any physical activity or other vigorous exercise.
- Begin any programme at a low level and gradually increase your activity.

Warming up correctly

Regardless of your age or level of fitness, you are at risk of straining yourself if you do not warm-up correctly. The programme outlined here includes an automatic warm-up method that depends upon both the arrangement in order of the exercises and the way in which they are carried out.

They begin with a stretching and then loosening exercise involving large muscles. This is to be done quite slowly and gently at first, and then gradually it increases in both speed and intensity.

An example can be seen in Exercise 1. At first you are not expected to be able to touch the floor, just to push down as far as you feel able to do without causing strain. Each time this is repeated the aim is to push just a little further. After two minutes at this you should be able to touch the floor with relative ease and quite quickly.

Why this exercise regime was developed

Research shows quite clearly that we all need exercise, whether young or old. In the modern world there are more and more labour-saving devices available both inside and outside the home. The result is that we lead a much more sedentary life than our predecessors.

Most of us claim we want to exercise and we know it is good for us; but we do not necessarily know how to go about it, how much to do, what kind of exercise to do and how we can judge progress.

Most exercise programmes require special equipment, often only available in a gym, which makes it difficult to exercise every day.

Also, considerable time is often required, which you may not have to spare.

It is therefore obvious that what is needed is a programme which overcomes these obstacles; one which does not require special equipment or long periods of time, and which also is easy to understand, where it is clear what to do next and how to measure your progress. This is such a programme, it requires no specialist equipment, it takes less than 15 minutes a day and needs only a small amount of space.

What is the exercise plan?

The plan has six charts arranged in order of difficulty. On each chart there are descriptions of five exercises. These should always be carried out in the same order each time, and keeping within the time limits set. As you move on from one chart to the next, the basic exercise will change just a little and will require just that bit more effort to carry out.

Level

Letters of the alphabet designate various levels of physical capacity.

Exercises

The first four exercises, Exercises 1, 2, 3 and 4, are illustrated and described later in the book. Column 1 is for the first exercise. The numbers found in each column represent the count, that is the number of times you need to be able to repeat this exercise in the allocated time. The fifth exercise is running on the spot. You can, however, make a substitution by running or walking for the required time instead of running in one place.

Time for each exercise

You will find the allocated time for each exercise at the bottom of the particular column. Exercises 1 to 5 together should be done in 11 minutes. At first you may find that there are some exercises which take a little longer, but there will also be those you complete in less than the time allocated. As long as the five exercises together take only 11 minutes that is fine.

14

Chart 3
Physical capacity rating scale

Level	Exercise					Minutes for:	
	1	2	3	4	5	1 mile run	2 mile walk
A+	30	32	47	24	550	8	25
A	30	31	45	22	540	8	25
A–	30	30	43	21	525	8	25
B+	28	28	41	20	510	8¼	28
B	28	27	39	19	500	8¼	26
B–	28	26	37	18	490	8¼	26
C+	26	25	35	17	480	8½	27
C	26	24	34	17	465	8½	27
C–	26	23	33	16	450	8½	27
D+	24	22	31	15	430	8¾	28
D	24	21	30	15	415	8¾	28
D–	24	20	29	15	400	8¾	29
Minutes for each exercise	2	1	1	1	6		

Age groups

12 Yrs maintains D+
13 Yrs maintains C+
14 yrs maintains B+
35-39 yrs maintains B
40-44 yrs maintains C
40-44 Yrs maintains A+
45-49 yrs maintains B

How far should you go?

How far you continue to progress with these exercises is determined by your age. These levels are based upon average levels of ability and of course there will always be those who can reach a higher level, as well as those who are not quite as fit. The goals given should therefore be treated as guides, rather than as absolutes to be reached at all costs.

Useful tips

- Do not give in to any desire to skip a day. This is likely to happen only at the beginning, because the further you progress, the more likely it is to fit into your routine and the more likely you are to enjoy your exercise time.

- As you progress through the course you may find that there are a few exercises which prove difficult for you to complete in 11 minutes. You will hit a mini-plateau, but do persist, day after day, and eventually you will be able to meet your target and move on.

- Some of you may find it hard to count all the steps needed in Exercise 5. It is so easy to lose count. Try dividing the number of steps needed by 75 or 50. Remember the answer. On a nearby surface, place a row of something such as coins or buttons equal to the answer. Do your first set of 75 or 50 steps and move one counter. Repeat until you have moved them all.

How to make a start

It is best if the exercises can be done at the same time each day, so choose a time when you are likely to have 11 minutes to spare on a regular basis, perhaps in the early morning, although you may prefer the evening or some other time, but whatever time you choose try hard to stick to it and *start today.*

Maximum rates of progress

- At least one day spent on each level for those aged 20
- At least two days at each level for those aged 20-29
- At least four days at each level for those aged 30-39
- At least seven days at each level for those aged 40-49

- At least eight days at each level for those aged 50-59
- At least 10 days at each level if you are 60 or over.

If you suffer any breathlessness, or you feel sore and stiff, especially if you are in one of the older age groups, slow up your rate of progress through the levels.

Note in the box available on each chart the recommended number of days needed on a level before progressing on to the next higher level.

Your progress

The Progress Chart is there to assist you in keeping a record of the progress you are making. Make a note of the starting and finishing date of each level. Also, write down your feelings about each level. Select an achievable aim and write this in on the bottom chart in the box labelled 'My Aim'. Your present measurements should be recorded on the start line. When you come to the end of each chart, make a note of your new measurements on the finish line. The changes may be quite subtle as fitness takes time and effort, so the results will not be amazing, but they will be positive. Combine these exercises with a balanced and sensible diet, and you will have success.

A note of caution

You may feel that you are already fairly fit and could start part way through the course. Don't give in to this temptation. You really do need to start at the beginning with Chart 1, Exercise 1. For the best results you should exercise each and every day. It may take you several months to get through to the final exercise, but after that you only need to exercise for three periods each week, and your fitness level will keep up.

If, for any reason, you do have to call a halt for a while, when you restart, do begin at a level which is a few below the one where you left off, even if your break has only been a short one. This is not about completing the course in a certain time, but completing it in as long as it takes you personally to reach optimum improvement and fitness.

To begin

Make a start at level D on the first chart. This requires the least physical ability. Each exercise should be repeated in the times given, or you could try five different exercises within a period of 11 minutes. Progress up the chart to level D, only if you are physically fit enough to do so. When you can do all the requirements for level A in the time allocated, then move on to Chart 2. Progress until you reach the maximum level expected for your age group, for example if you are 35 this fits into the age group 35-39 and you should continue to level B on the third chart.

Chart 1

Chart 1
Physical capacity rating scale

Level	Exercise					Minutes for:	
	1	2	3	4	5	½ mile run	1 mile walk
A+	20	18	22	13	400	5½	17
A	18	17	20	12	375	5½	17
A–	16	15	18	11	335	5½	17
B+	14	13	16	9	320	6	18
B	12	12	14	8	305	6	18
B–	10	11	12	7	280	6	18
C+	8	9	10	6	260	6½	19
C	7	8	9	5	235	6½	19
C–	6	7	8	4	205	6½	19
D+	4	5	6	3	175	7	20
D	3	4	5	3	145	7½	21
D–	2	3	4	2	100	8	21
Minutes for each exercise	2	1	1	1	6		

Age Groups
6 yrs   maintains   B
7 yrs   maintains   A

My progress
Physical capacity rating scale

Level	Exercise					Minutes for:	
	1	2	3	4	5	1 mile run	1 mile walk
A+							
A							
A–							
B+							
B							
B–							
C+							
C							
C–							
D+							
D							
D–							
Minutes for each exercise	2	1	1	1	6		

	Date	Height	Weight
My aim			
Start			
Finish			

1 Toe touching

Stand with your feet apart and your arms up. Now, bend over so that you can reach the floor with your fingertips and then rise and stretch backwards. Keep your legs straight, but do not strain.

CHART 1

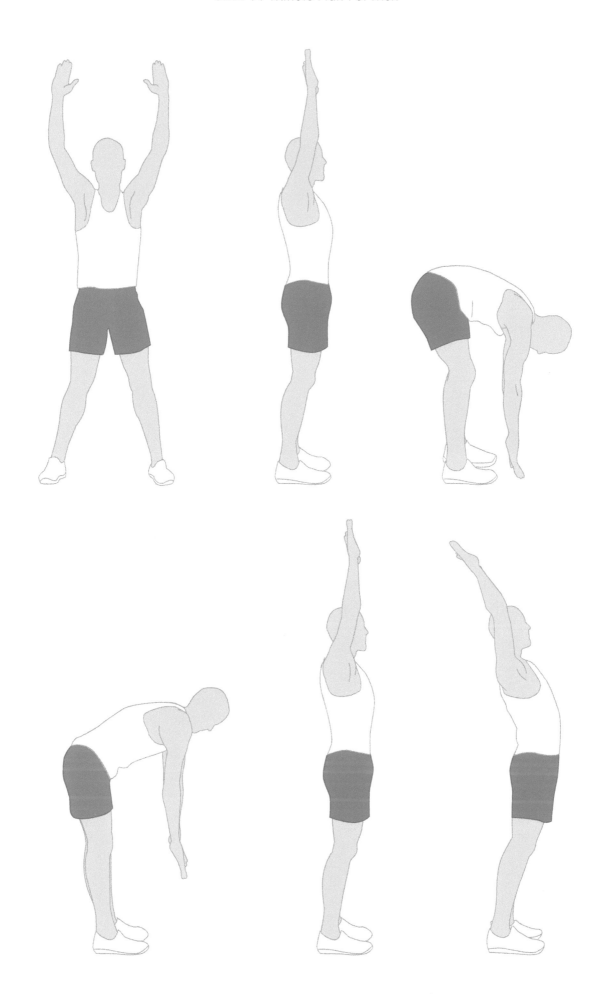

2 *Sit-ups*

Lie on your back with your arms by your sides and with your feet about six inches apart. Sit up enough to enable you to see your heels. Your legs must remain straight and your head and shoulders must lift up from the floor. Return to the start position.

CHART 1

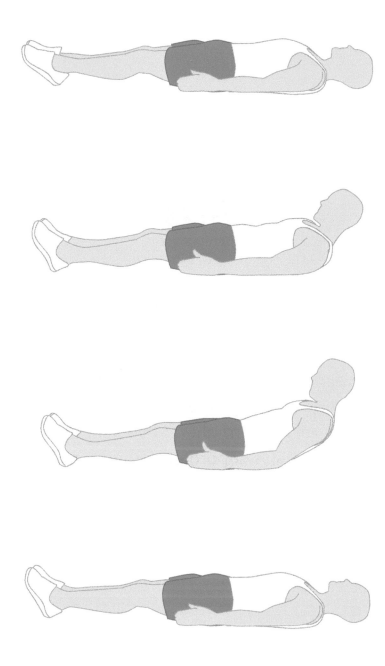

3 Leg raising

Lie on your front with your arms at your sides and with your palms under your thighs. Raise your head together with one leg. Return to the start position. Repeat with the other leg. Count once when the second leg is returned to the floor. Your legs must remain straight and you should lift the leg up so that it is separated from the palm.

CHART 1

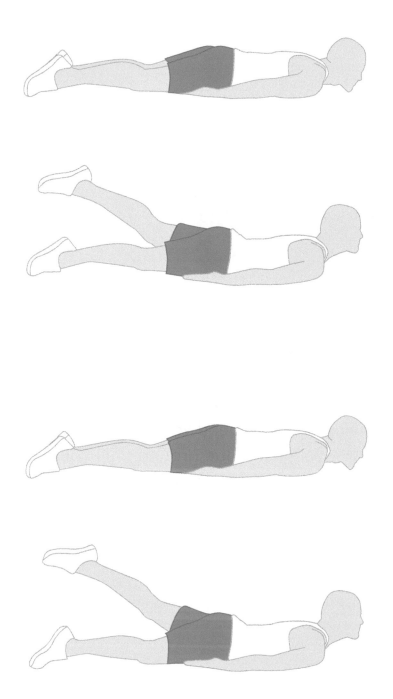

4 Push-ups

Lie on your front with your hands placed under your shoulders and with your palms down on the floor. Keeping your knees on the floor, lift up your upper body by straightening your arms to their full extent. Bend your arms once more to lower yourself to the ground until your chest comes back into contact with the floor.

CHART 1

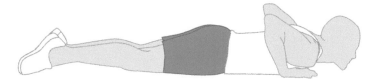

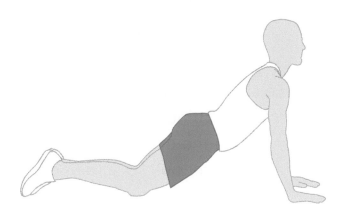

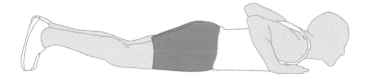

5 *The stationary run and scissor steps*

You count one step each time your left foot leaves the ground. You need to lift each foot at least 4 inches above the ground. Once you have counted 75 steps, carry out 10 scissor steps.

Scissor steps

Stand with your right leg placed forward and your other leg placed behind you. Your left arm should be extended at shoulder height forwards and with your right one extended behind you. Now jump, reversing these positions.

CHART 1

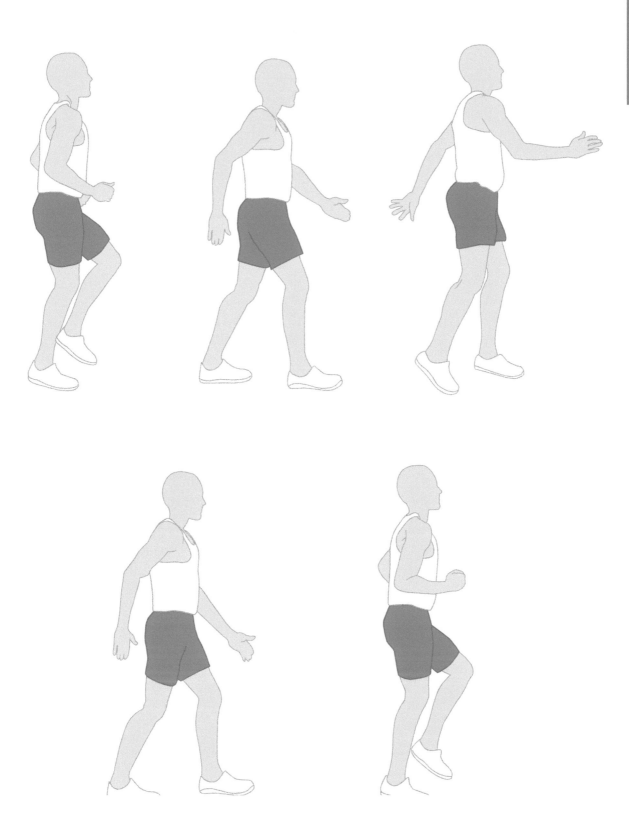

Chart 2

Chart 2
Physical capacity rating scale

Level	Exercise					Minutes for:	
	1	2	3	4	5	1 mile run	2 mile walk
A+	30	23	33	20	500	9	30
A	29	21	31	19	485	9	31
A–	28	20	29	18	470	9	32
B+	26	18	27	17	455	9½	33
B	24	17	25	16	445	9½	33
B–	22	16	23	15	440	9½	33
C+	20	15	21	14	425	10	34
C	19	14	19	13	410	10	34
C–	18	13	17	12	395	10	34
D+	16	12	15	11	380	10½	35
D	15	11	14	10	360	10½	35
D–	14	10	13	9	335	10½	35
Minutes for each exercise	2	1	1	1	6		

Age Groups

8 yrs	maintains	D–
9 yrs	maintains	C–
10 yrs	maintains	B–
11 yrs	maintains	A–
45-49 yrs	maintains	A+
50-60 yrs	maintains	C+

My progress
Physical capacity rating scale

Level	Exercise					Minutes for:	
	1	2	3	4	5	1 mile run	2 mile walk
A+							
A							
A–							
B+							
B							
B–							
C+							
C							
C–							
D+							
D							
D–							
Minutes for each exercise	2	1	1	1	6		

	Date	Height	Weight
My aim			
Start			
Finish			

1 **Floor touch and bounce**

Stand with your feet astride and with your arms raised upwards. Bend and touch the floor between your feet, bounce up part way and then touch again, before stretching and extending your back to the rear. Keep your knees as straight as you can, but do not strain to do so.

CHART 2

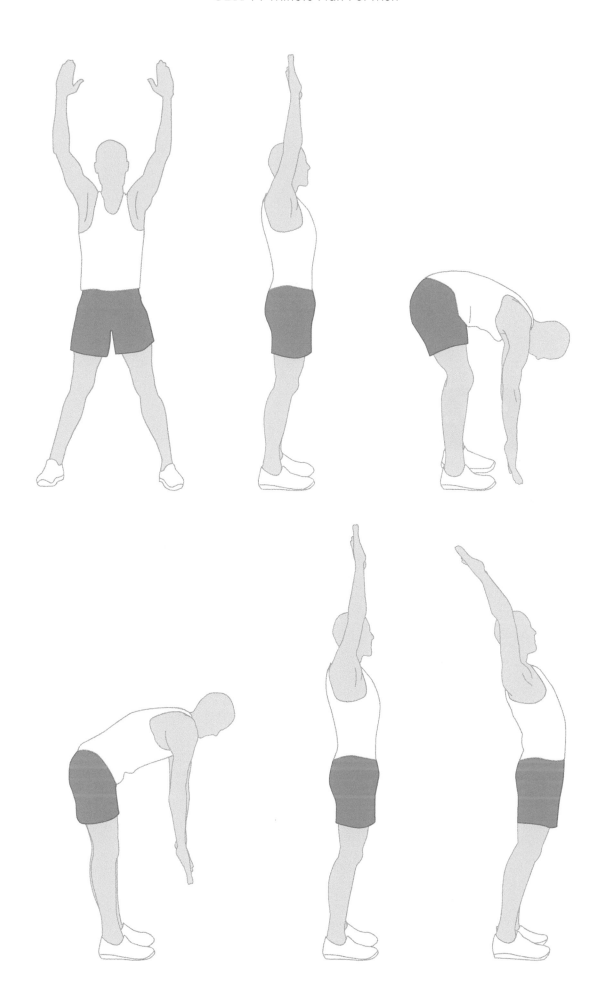

2 Sit-ups

Lie flat on the floor. Your arms should be at your side and your legs straight. Sit up so that your back is now in a vertical position. Keep your feet on the floor. You may find it useful to hook your feet underneath a chair, you should allow your knees to bend a little.

CHART 2

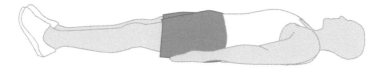

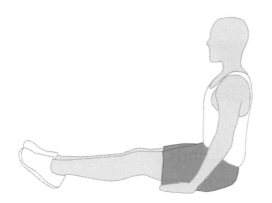

3 *Front pull-ups*

Lie face down. Your hands should be placed beneath your thighs. Raise your legs together with your head and shoulders. Your legs should remain in a straight position and your thighs should clear your hands.

CHART 2

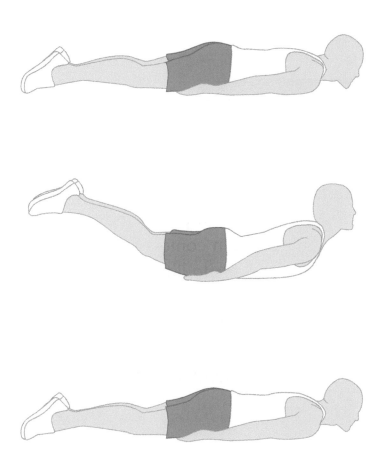

4 Push-ups

Lie face down with your hands placed under your shoulders and with your hands turned so that your palms are in contact with the floor. Push up on your arms to lift your body up from the floor until only your toes and palms are in contact with the floor. You should keep your back in a straight line. Return to the first position so that your chest is in contact with the floor.

CHART 2

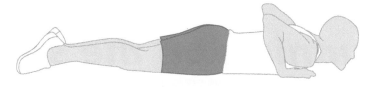

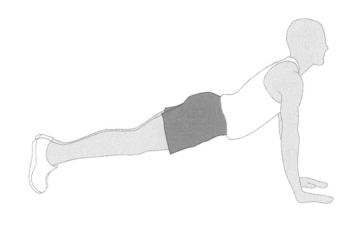

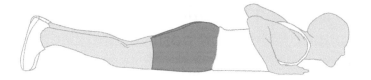

5 Running on the spot and astride jumps

Each time you lift your left foot up from the floor counts as one. Your feet should be lifted at least 4 inches up from the floor. After you have counted to 75, carry out 10 astride jumps.

Astride jumps

Your feet should be placed closely next to each other, and your arms should be placed alongside your sides. Take a jump with your arms held out straight to the sides slightly above the shoulder line. You should land with your feet astride. Jump again back to the start position and count one.

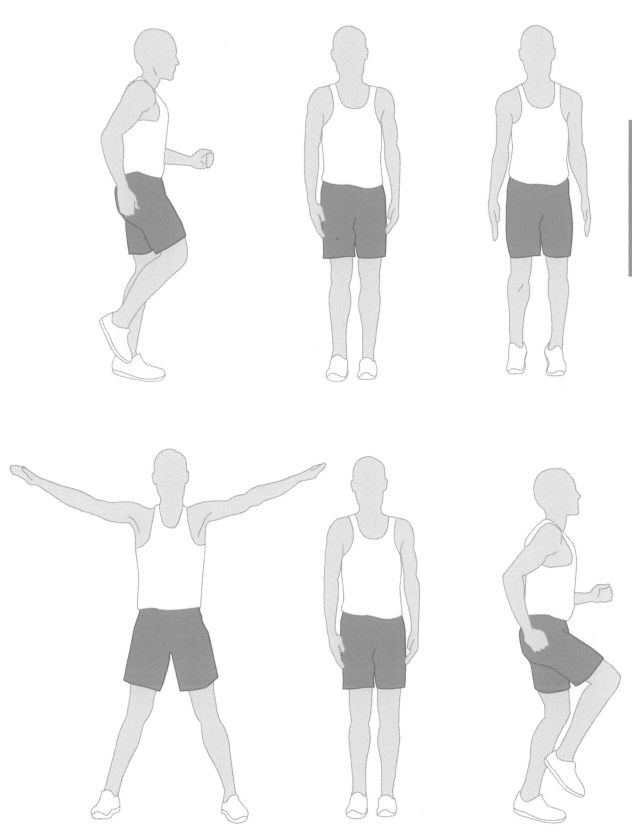

CHART 2

Chart 3

Chart 3
Physical capacity rating scale

Level	Exercise					Minutes for:	
	1	2	3	4	5	1 mile run	2 mile walk
A+	30	32	47	24	550	8	25
A	30	31	45	22	540	8	25
A–	30	30	43	21	525	8	25
B+	28	28	41	20	510	8¼	28
B	28	27	39	19	500	8¼	26
B–	28	26	37	18	490	8¼	26
C+	26	25	35	17	480	8½	27
C	26	24	34	17	465	8½	27
C–	26	23	33	16	450	8½	27
D+	24	22	31	15	430	8¾	28
D	24	21	30	15	415	8¾	28
D–	24	20	29	15	400	8¾	29
Minutes for each exercise	2	1	1	1	6		

Age Groups

12 yrs	maintains	D+
13 yrs	maintains	C+
14 yrs	maintains	B+
35-39 yrs	maintains	B
40-44 yrs	maintains	C

Flying Crew

40-44 yrs	maintains	A+
45-49 yrs	maintains	B

My progress
Physical capacity rating scale

Level	Exercise					Minutes for:	
	1	**2**	**3**	**4**	**5**	**1 mile run**	**2 mile walk**
A+							
A							
A–							
B+							
B							
B–							
C+							
C							
C–							
D+							
D							
D–							
Minutes for each exercise	2	1	1	1	6		

	Date	Height	Weight
My aim			
Start			
Finish			

1 Floor touchdown

You should stand with your arms up and your feet astride. Bend so that you can touch the floor 6 inches to the left of your left foot. Bounce and touch the floor again, this time between your feet and then outside your right foot, before standing up and bending back as far as you can. This counts as one. When you reach the halfway point in your count, reverse your directions, that is touch the right side first. Do not struggle to keep your knees in a straight position.

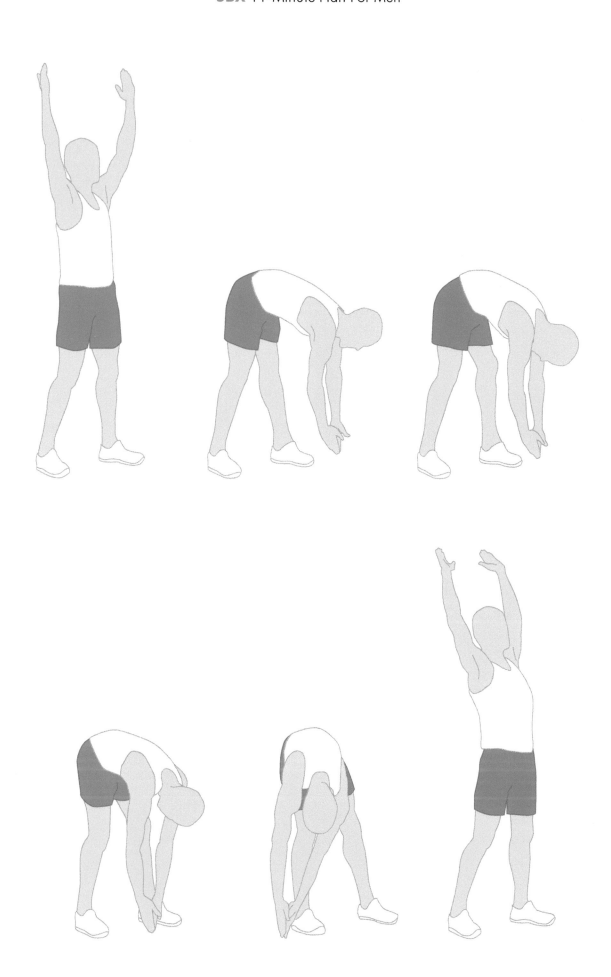

CHART 3

2 Sit-ups

Lie down on your back with your hands clasped at the back of your head. Your legs should be straight and with your heels six inches apart. Keeping your feet on the floor, perhaps hooked below a chair, sit up into the vertical position.

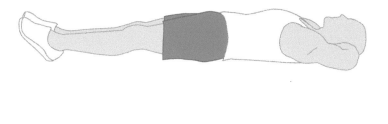

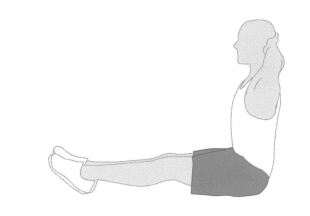

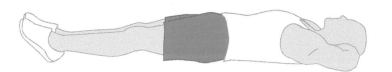

CHART 3

3 Lift-ups

Lie on your front with your hands clasped behind your lower back. Now lift up both your head and upper body, as well as your legs and feet, as far as you can. Your legs should remain straight and your thighs should be raised above the floor. Return to the first position.

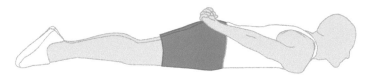

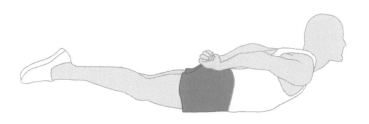

CHART 3

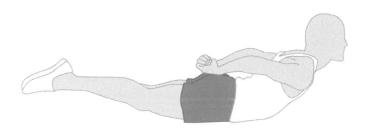

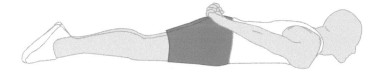

4 Push-ups with touches

Lie on your front with your hands placed under your shoulders and with your palms placed down to touch the floor. Touch the floor with your chin in front of your hands. Next, touch the floor with your brow and then straighten your arms to raise your body. These are three distinct movements which count as one.

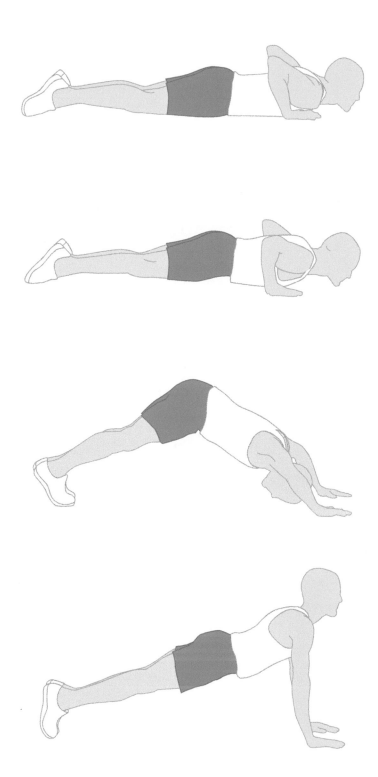

CHART 3

Running on the spot and half knee bending

Run on the spot, lifting each foot at least 4 inches up. Each time your left foot returns to the floor you can count one. After a count of 75, carry out 10 half knee bends.

Half knee bending

With your feet placed close together, place your hands on your hips and bend your knees to create an angle of about 110 degrees. Straighten until you are erect, and then lift your heels up from the floor. Your back should remain straight and your feet should not leave contact with the floor. Return to the start position.

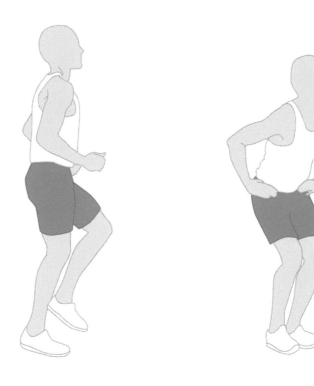

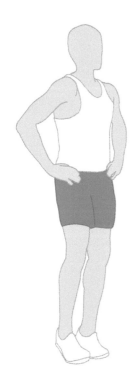

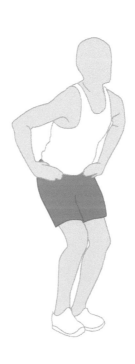

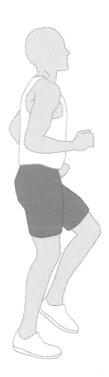

CHART 3

Chart 4

Chart 4
Physical capacity rating scale

Level	Exercise					Minutes for:	
	1	2	3	4	5	1 mile run	2 mile walk
A+	30	22	50	42	400	7	19
A	30	22	49	40	395	7	19
A–	30	22	49	37	390	7	19
B+	28	21	47	34	380	7¼	20
B	28	21	46	32	375	7¼	20
B–	28	21	46	30	365	7¼	20
C+	26	19	44	28	355	7½	21
C	26	19	43	26	345	7½	21
C–	26	19	43	24	335	7½	21
D+	24	18	41	21	325	7¾	23
D	24	18	40	19	315	7¾	23
D–	24	18	40	17	300	7¾	23
Minutes for each exercise	2	1	1	1	6		

Age Groups

15 yrs	maintains	D–
16-17 yrs	maintains	C+
25-29 yrs	maintains	A+
30-34 yrs	maintains	C–

Flying Crew

30-34 yrs	maintains	B
35-39 yrs	maintains	C–

My progress
Physical capacity rating scale

Level	Exercise					Minutes for:	
	1	2	3	4	5	1 mile run	2 mile walk
A+							
A							
A–							
B+							
B							
B–							
C+							
C							
C–							
D+							
D							
D–							
Minutes for each exercise	2	1	1	1	6		

	Date	Height	Weight
My aim			
Start			
Finish			

1 *Floor touching with arm circling*

Stand with your feet placed widely apart and your arms pointing to the sky. Bend down so that you can touch the floor outside your left foot, followed by touching between your feet and then towards the right. Do not try too hard to keep your knees straight. Stand up and bend yourself backwards. Keep your arms raised and describe a circle. After half your count, reverse the direction of your moves.

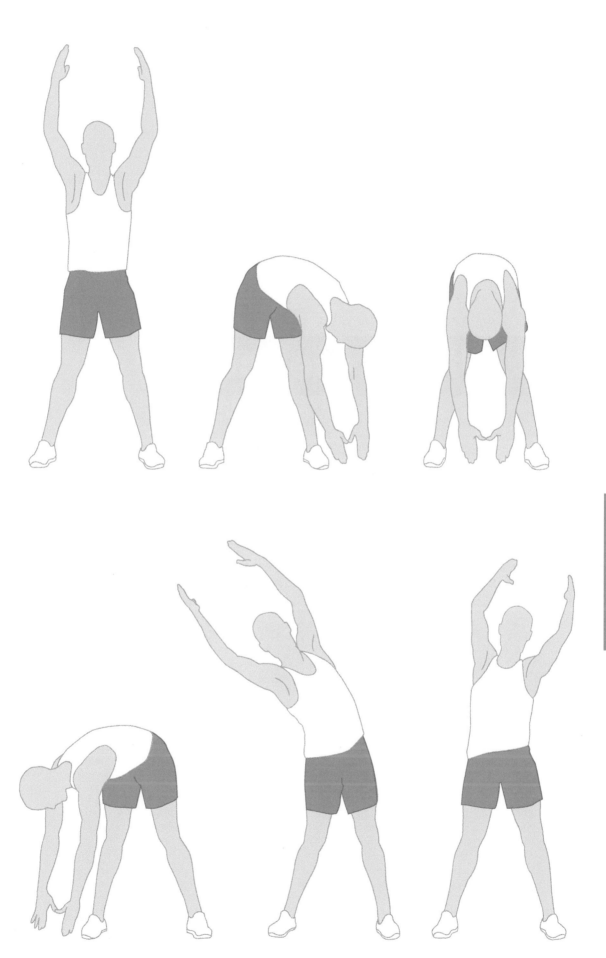

CHART 4

2 *Sitting toe touch*

You should lie down on your back with your arms
back above your head. Your legs should be straight
out and your feet close together. Keeping your
arms and legs straight, and perhaps hooking your
feet under a chair to prevent them rising, sit up
so that you can touch your toe tips. Your arms
should be kept close to the sides of your head
throughout. Lie back down and count one.

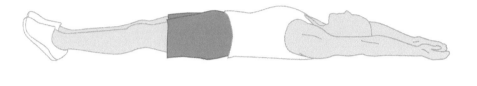

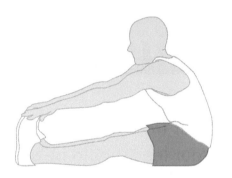

CHART 4

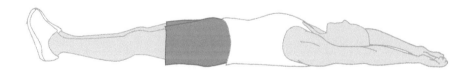

3 *Double front lift*

Lie down on your front with your arms stretched out
to the sides. Your legs should be stretched out and
straight. Lift your head, upper body and legs up
from the floor as high as you possibly can with arms
swinging backwards. Return to the starting position.

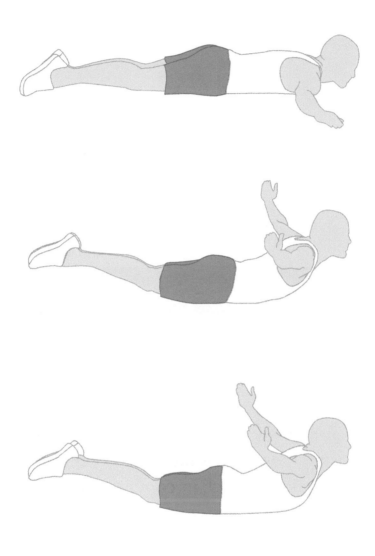

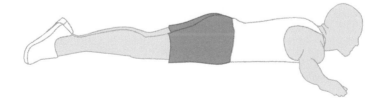

CHART 4

4 Push-ups from the head

Lie on your front with your hands placed palms down on the floor about a foot each side of your head. Straighten your arms completely to raise your body as high as is possible. Relax and lower yourself until your chest is back in contact with the floor.

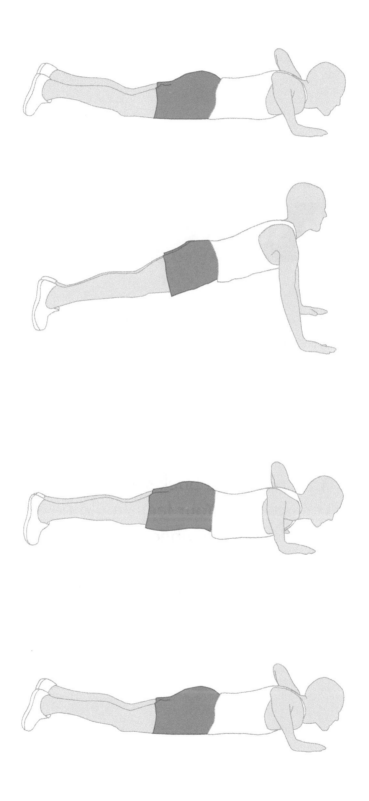

CHART 4

5 Running on the spot with semi-squats

Run on the spot, but this time raise your knees waist high with each step. Do 10 semi-squat jumps after each 75 steps.

Semi-squat jumps

Half crouch with your hands palm down on your knees. Your arms and back should remain as straight as possible. Your feet should be placed so that one foot is slightly ahead of the other. Keeping your body straight, jump up so that your feet are raised above the floor. In the short time before you land, once more reverse the positions of your feet. Crouch again and repeat nine more times.

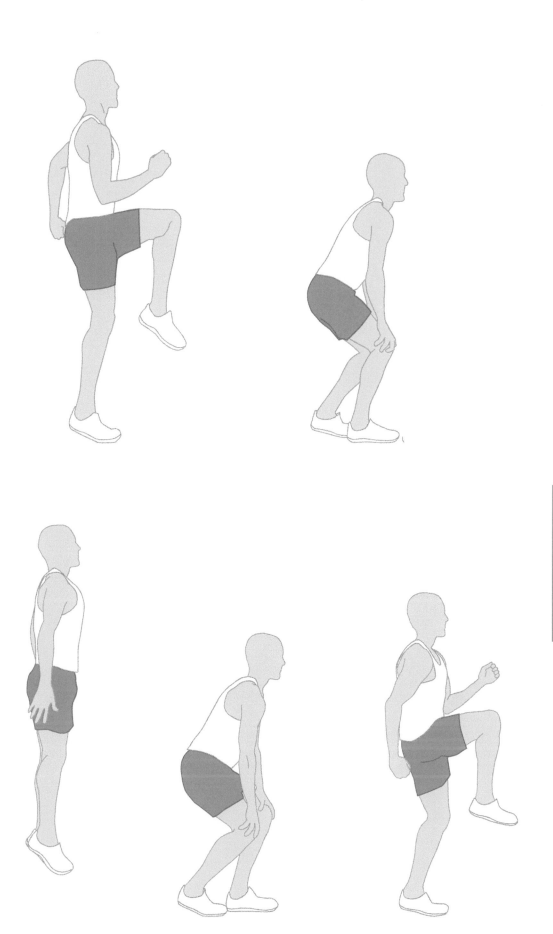

CHART 4

Chart 5

Chart 5
Physical capacity rating scale

Level	Exercise					Mins:Secs for
	1	2	3	4	5	1 mile run
A+	30	40	50	44	500	6:00
A	30	39	49	43	485	6:06
A–	30	38	48	42	475	6:09
B+	28	36	47	40	465	6:12
B	28	35	46	39	455	6:15
B–	28	34	45	38	445	6:21
C+	26	32	44	36	435	6:27
C	26	31	43	35	420	6:33
C–	26	30	42	34	410	6:39
D+	24	28	41	32	400	6:45
D	24	27	40	31	385	6:51
D–	24	26	39	30	375	7:00
Minutes for each exercise	2	1	1	1	6	

Age Groups
 18–25 yrs   maintains   C

Flying Crew
Under 25 yrs   maintains   B+
25-29 yrs   maintains   D+

My progress
Physical capacity rating scale

Level	Exercise					Mins:Secs for
	1	2	3	4	5	1 mile run
A+						
A						
A–						
B+						
B						
B–						
C+						
C						
C–						
D+						
D						
D–						
Minutes for each exercise	2	1	1	1	6	

	Date	Height	Weight
My aim			
Start			
Finish			

1 *Striding floor touch*

Place your feet astride and stand up straight. Your arms should be held straight above your head with your hands clasped. Firstly, touch the floor to the left of your feet, then between them, and thirdly to the right. Stand and circle your body back as far as possible. Do not worry too much about the straightness of your knees. After half the counts, reverse your directions.

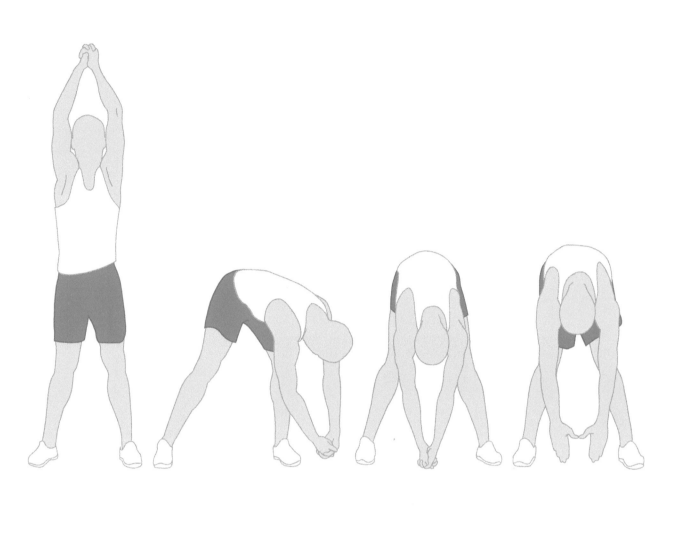

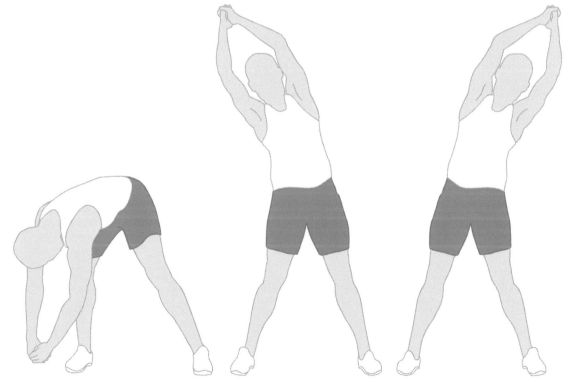

CHART 5

2 Sit and twist

Lying on your back with your legs kept straight and your feet close together, clasp your hands behind your head. Sit erect and bend up your knees. Twist from the waist so that you can touch your left knee with the tip of your right elbow. For this move count one. Repeat, but alternate your direction. When your knee and elbow come into contact your feet should be up off the floor. Return to the first position between sit-ups.

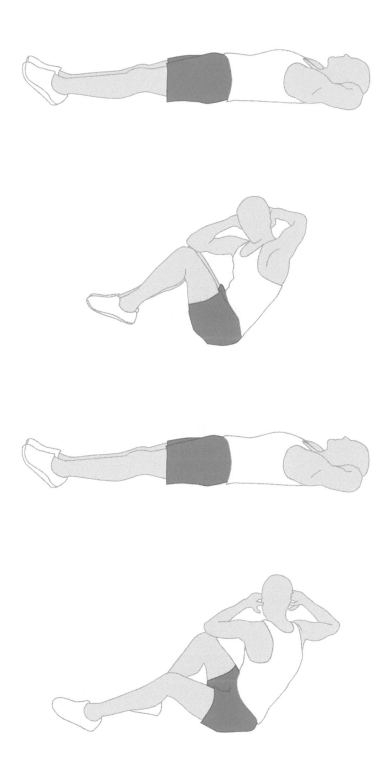

CHART 5

81

3 *Frontal double lift*

Lie face down with your arms extended up past the sides of your head. Keeping your legs straight, lift them up as high as you can, while at the same time lifting your arms, head and upper torso, so that you are lying on your pelvis and lower abdomen. Return to the flat and count one.

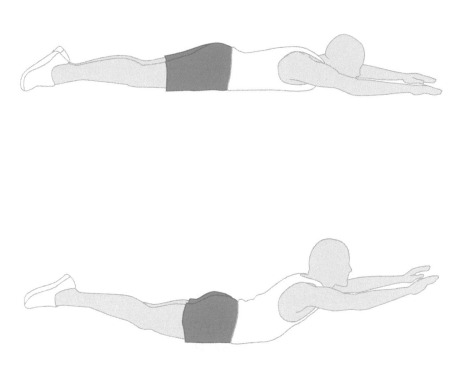

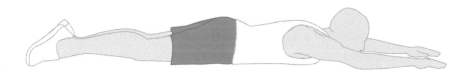

CHART 5

4 Push-up and clap

Lie down on your front. Your hands should be below your shoulders and your palms should be placed flat on the floor. Push upwards by extending your arms fully. Clap your hands very quickly before lying down once more. Your body should stay in a straight line at all times.

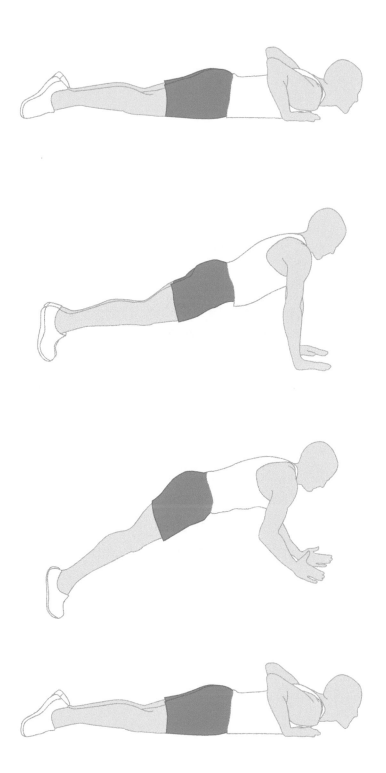

CHART 5

Running on the spot with half spreadeagle jumps

Run on the spot, lifting the knees as high as your waist each time. Count one every time your second foot returns into contact with the floor. After a count of 75, carry out half spreadeagle jumps to a count of 10.

Half spreadeagle jumps

With your feet close together, drop down into half crouch. Your hands should be on your knees and with your arms kept straight. Jump upwards so that your feet are astride and your arms swing upwards. Return to your first position. Your feet should be at least your shoulder width apart, before coming back to land close together.

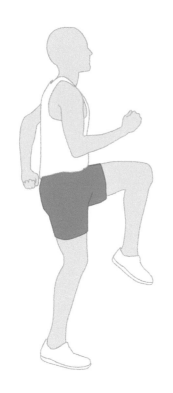
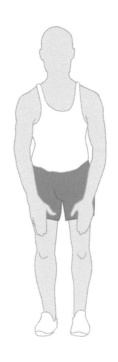

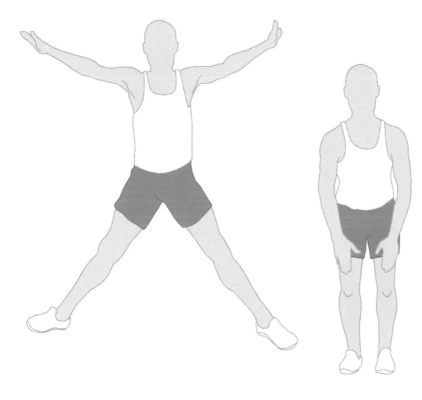
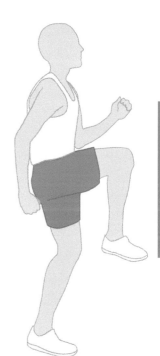

CHART 5

Chart 6

Chart 6
Physical capacity rating scale

Level	Exercise					Mins:Secs for
	1	2	3	4	5	1 mile run
A+	30	50	40	40	600	5:00
A	30	48	39	39	580	5:03
A–	30	47	38	38	555	5:09
B+	28	45	37	36	530	5:12
B	28	44	36	35	525	5:18
B–	28	43	35	34	515	5:24
C+	26	41	34	32	505	5:27
C	26	40	33	31	495	5:33
C–	26	39	32	30	485	5:39
D+	24	37	31	28	475	5:45
D	24	36	30	27	460	5:51
D–	24	35	29	26	450	6:00
Minutes for each exercise	2	1	1	1	6	

Physical capacities in this chart are usually found only in champion athletes

My progress
Physical capacity rating scale

Level	Exercise					Mins:Secs for
	1	2	3	4	5	1 mile run
A+						
A						
A–						
B+						
B						
B–						
C+						
C						
C–						
D+						
D						
D–						
Minutes for each exercise	2	1	1	1	6	

	Date	Height	Weight
My aim			
Start			
Finish			

1 *Floor touch with*
reverse hand clasp

Stand with your feet astride. Your hands should be clasped high above your head with their positions reversed. Bend so that you can touch the floor to one side of your feet, then in the centre and thirdly to the other side. Stand back up and bend your torso backwards and circle. Your hands should stay in the reverse clasp position. After you have reached the half count reverse your direction.

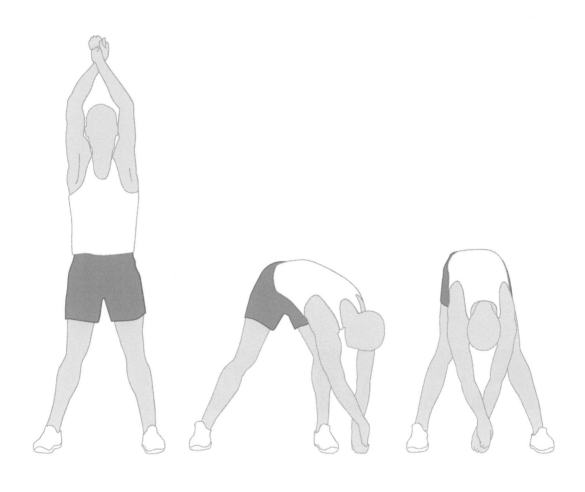

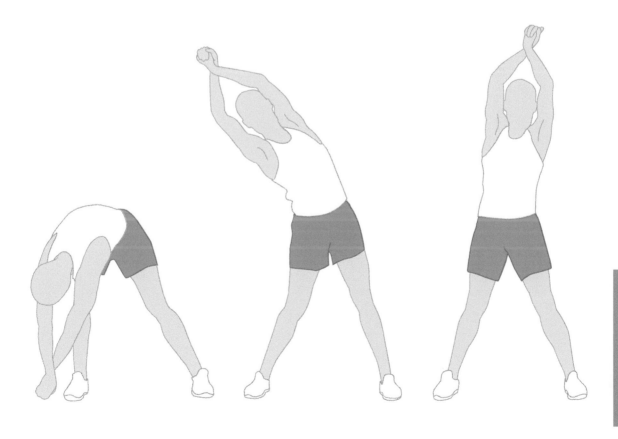

CHART 6

93

2 *Sit-up with pike*

Lie down on your back with your arms placed straight above your head. Sit up so that you can touch your toes with your legs in the pike position. Your feet should be kept close together and your legs should clear the floor each time. Return to the rest position and count one.

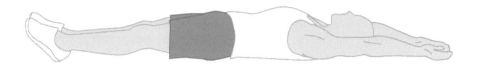

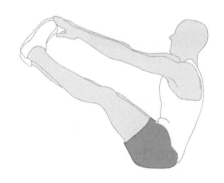

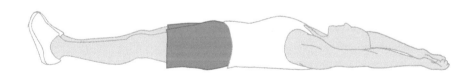

CHART 6

3 *Double lift*

Lie down on your front with your arms placed in a straight line above your head. Lift up your legs, head and upper body as high as possible and at the same time. Press up once. Your limbs should be kept straight and your legs and chest should clear the floor completely. Return to start position.

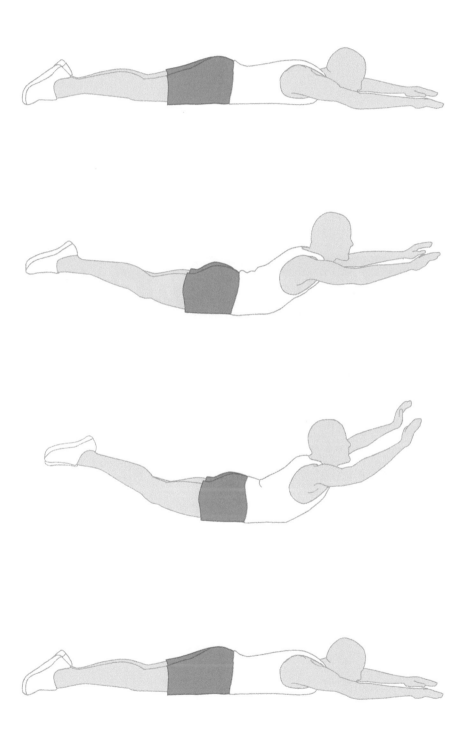

CHART 6

4 Push-ups with chest slap

Lie on your front with your palms flat on the ground under your shoulders. Push up to extend your arms fully and then slap your chest so that this can be heard before lowering yourself. Your body should be kept in a straight line at all times.

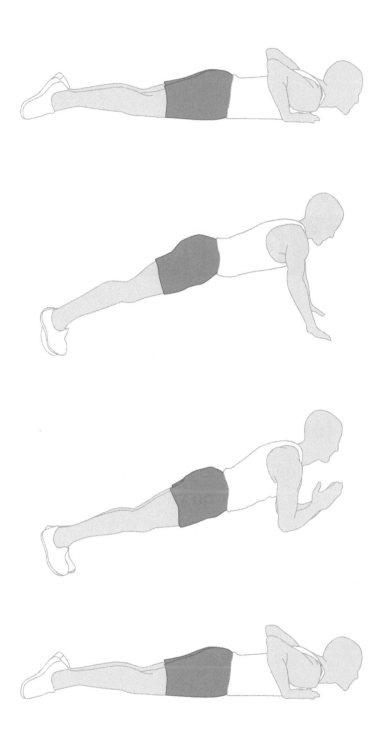

CHART 6

99

5 *Running on the spot with jack jumps*

Run, lifting your knees up to waist height. Each time your left foot lands, count one. After 75 steps, carry out 10 jack jumps.

Jack jumps

Place your feet close together and bend your knees so that you can sit back on your heels and your fingertips should touch the floor in front of you. Jump upwards, with legs to the side, raising your legs to waist height. Keep your legs straight and touch your toes mid-jump.

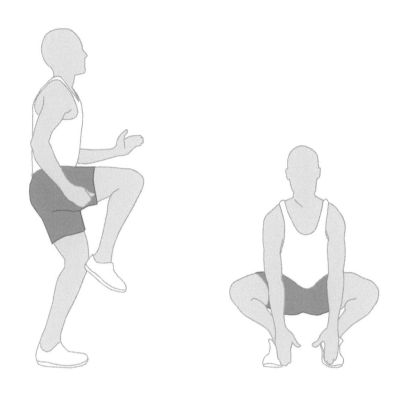

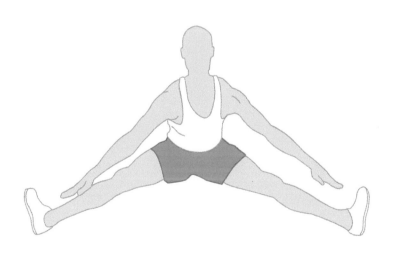

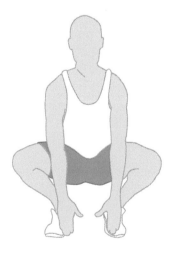

CHART 6